LUNG SURGERY HEALING FOODS

Complete Guide Unlocking The Secrets Of
Nutrition To Rapid Healing After Surgery
Success, Nourishing Meal Plans, Recipes, Tips
For Optimal Health Wellness)

DR. ALLAN FREDA

Contents

This complete guide gives you information on how to eat well after surgery to help your body heal and stay healthy in the long run. People who read it will find a lot of mending recipes, personalised meal plans, and expert tips that were put together to help the body recover from lung surgery. This book is an essential resource for people who have just been diagnosed because it contains tried-and-true methods that will help them find their way to better health and vitality.

INTRODUCTION

How to Know How Important Food Is for Lung Surgery Recovery

Nutrition is very important for getting better after surgery on the lungs. To heal properly, the body needs a wide range of nutrients, especially after a treatment that can be hard on the body. To repair tissues and cells, good nutrition is important. It also boosts the immune system, lowers the risk of getting sick, and improves general health.

People who are having surgery on their lungs need to make sure they eat a balanced diet because it can help them heal faster and have better results after surgery. You can't say enough about how important diet is in this situation because it directly affects the body's ability to heal and get stronger.

When you're recovering from lung surgery, the first thing you should do is focus on what you eat.

For newly diagnosed patients to get through their healing process successfully, they need a complete guide to the best diet after surgery.

Not only does this guide stress the importance of certain healing foods, but it also gives you ideas on how to plan your meals and includes healing recipes, meal plans, and health advice from experts for long-term wellness.

By learning about the importance of nutrition in recovery after surgery and making healthy eating a regular habit, patients can speed up the healing process and improve their general health.

How Healing Foods Help People Get Better After Lung Surgery

Healing foods are very important for getting better after lung surgery because they give the body the nutrients it needs to mend tissues, keep the immune system healthy, and stay healthy overall. There are a lot of vitamins, minerals, antioxidants, and other bioactive substances in these foods that help the body heal and lower inflammation.

By adding healing foods to your diet, you can speed up your recovery, ease your symptoms, and improve your quality of life after surgery. Learning about the specific foods that your body needs to heal and adding them to your meals can make a big difference in how quickly you recover after lung surgery.

Adding nutrient-dense foods to your diet after surgery is very important for speeding up the healing process. There are a lot of vitamins, minerals, and other nutrients in these foods that help the body heal and improve health in general. Fruits, veggies, lean proteins, whole grains, and healthy fats are all examples of foods that are high in nutrients. These foods give the body the building blocks it needs to heal tissues, boost the immune system, and lower the risk of problems while the body heals. People who are having surgery on their lungs can speed up their healing and improve their general health by focusing on nutrient-rich foods.

Recipes that will help you heal after lung surgery

It can be very helpful to make healing recipes that are specific to the nutritional needs of people who are suffering from lung surgery. These recipes are meant to be healthy, simple to stomach, and full of ingredients that help the body heal.

Foods that are good for you, like leafy greens, colorful veggies, lean proteins, and whole grains, are often used in healing recipes. Also, they usually don't have a lot of salt, sugar, or bad fats, which is good for your heart and general health. Patients who have had lung surgery can feed their bodies and speed up their recovery by making and eating healing recipes.

Food plans for long-term health

People who are healing from lung surgery need to make meal plans for long-term health. The goal of these meal plans is to give you a healthy, well-balanced diet that helps you heal and stay healthy generally. When someone is recovering from lung surgery, their meal plans usually include a lot of healthy foods, like fruits, veggies, lean proteins, whole grains, and healthy fats. Additionally, they think about any dietary needs or limits to make sure that people can enjoy tasty and filling meals while they are getting better. Patients can develop healthy eating habits that will help them stay healthy and speed up their recovery by sticking to well-thought-out meal plans.

Expert Advice on the Best Ways to Eat and Recover

Along with healing foods, meal plans, and recipes, adding expert advice on how to eat well and recover can speed up the healing process after lung surgery. Some of these tips could be about how to control your portions, stay hydrated, take supplements, and deal with certain surgery-related complaints or side effects. Talking to a qualified dietitian or nutritionist can also give you useful information and personalised suggestions to help with your recovery and long-term health. People who have had lung surgery can speed up the healing process and improve their quality of life by following the food and lifestyle suggestions of experts.

 diet is very important for getting better after lung surgery. People can improve their general health and speed up their healing process by learning about the importance of healing foods, meal planning, and getting professional help. People can support their best recovery and long-term health after surgery by eating nutrient-dense foods, following healing recipes and meal plans, and getting advice from experts. This complete guide is very helpful for people who have just been identified because it gives them the tools and information, they need to manage their healing process well and improve their health.

Disclaimer

The information in this book is for informational purposes only and should not replace professional medical advice, diagnosis, or treatment. Always consult your physician or a qualified health provider regarding any medical concerns. Do not disregard professional medical advice or delay seeking it based on information in this book.

The author does not endorse or have affiliations with any mentioned entities. References are for informational purposes only.

Consult your healthcare provider before making dietary or lifestyle changes, especially during recovery from surgery, as individual needs vary.

Results may vary, and the information provided is not guaranteed to produce specific outcomes.

By reading this book, you acknowledge and agree to consult your healthcare provider before implementing any information herein.

For further guidance, consult your healthcare provider or reputable medical websites for reliable information on surgery recovery diets.

CHAPTER 1
GETTING READY FOR SURGERY

Before any surgery, including lung surgery, it's important to make sure the body is ready so that it can heal and recover as quickly as possible. Preparing for surgery includes many things, such as eating right, drinking enough water, and supporting your nervous system. By focusing on these things, people can make themselves stronger, reduce problems, and help their bodies heal faster after surgery.

Advice on what to eat before surgery on the lungs

A lot of what you eat affects how well your body gets ready for surgery. People who are going to have lung surgery should follow certain dietary guidelines to improve their health and make their body better able to handle the process. For good health and a stronger immune system, you need to eat a healthy diet full of nutrients like vitamins, minerals, protein, and antioxidants. Adding a range of fruits, veggies, whole grains, lean proteins, and healthy fats to your diet can give your body the nutrients it needs to heal damaged tissues and boost your immune system.

Also, in the days before surgery, it's important to stay away from things that can make inflammation worse or cause digestive problems. You should limit foods that are high in sugar, refined carbs, saturated fats, and salt because they can make inflammation worse and make it harder for the body to heal. Focus on eating whole, nutrient-dense foods that are good for you and help you stay healthy.

Along with eating a healthy diet, some people may benefit from adding vitamins and minerals to their diet that are known to help the immune system work better and speed up the healing process. Some nutrients, like vitamin C, zinc, vitamin D, and omega-3 fatty acids, have been shown to help the body heal faster after surgery and lower the risk of problems. But it's important to talk to a doctor before taking any new supplements because they might not work well with other medicines or have bad effects.

Overall, eating right before lung surgery can help get the body ready for the stress of the treatment, speed up the healing process, and make things better.

Foods that will make your immune system stronger

For the best healing and recovery after lung surgery, you need a strong immune system. People know that some foods can help boost the immune system and make the body's defenses stronger against illness and inflammation. Adding these things to your diet before surgery can help your immune system get ready and make it better able to handle the stress of the procedure.

Fruits and veggies that are high in vitamins, minerals, and antioxidants are one type of food that can help your immune system. Citrus fruits, berries, leafy greens, bell peppers, and cruciferous veggies are all great places to get vitamin C, vitamin A, and other important nutrients that help the immune system work. These foods protect the body from oxidative stress and help make more white blood cells, which are very important for fighting off diseases.

Adding foods that are high in probiotics to your diet can also help keep your gut bacteria healthy, which is linked to immune function. Fermented foods like yogurt, kefir, sauerkraut, kimchi, and others have good bacteria in them that help keep the microbiome healthy and boost immune health. These foods can help lower the risk of getting infections after surgery and speed up the mending process.

Also, eating foods that are high in protein is important for keeping your immune system healthy and helping tissues heal.

Proteins that are low in fat, like those found in chicken, fish, tofu, beans, and nuts, help cells grow and keep the immune system strong. Getting enough protein before surgery can help the body heal faster by giving it the tools it needs to fix damaged tissues.

Overall, eating a lot of immune-boosting foods before lung surgery can help make the body's defenses stronger, lower the risk of problems, and speed up the healing and recovery process.

How to Stay Hydrated and Get Ready for Surgery

Staying hydrated is important for your health and well-being in general, but it's especially important before surgery. Staying well-hydrated is an important part of getting your body ready for surgery and helping it heal as quickly as possible afterward. Dehydration can hurt many body processes, like circulation, the immune system, and tissue repair. That's why it's very important to stay properly hydrated before lung surgery.

People should try to drink a lot of water in the days before surgery to make sure they are properly hydrated. Water is the best way to stay hydrated because it has no calories and is needed to keep the body's fluid balance. You should try to drink eight glasses of water every day, or more if you are very busy or live somewhere hot.

In addition to water, herbal teas, coconut water, and sports drinks that are high in electrolytes can also help you stay hydrated and replace lost fluids. Avoid drinking too many sugary or caffeinated drinks because they can make you pee a lot, which can make you dehydrated.

It's particularly important to stay hydrated on the day of surgery, since the body may have to fast and drink less fluids before the procedure. Dehydration can make complications more likely during surgery and make it take longer to heal afterward. It's important to stay well-hydrated before surgery and follow your doctor's advice about how long you should fast and how much fluid you should drink.

general, staying properly hydrated before lung surgery is important for your general health, for getting the best results from the surgery, and for speeding up your healing and recovery. By making sure they stay hydrated and eat right, people can get their bodies ready for surgery and make it easier for them to handle the stress of the process.

CHAPTER 2

WHAT YOU NEED AFTER SURGERY

How to Eat After Surgery: An Introduction

When someone has surgery on their lungs, their body goes through a lot of stress and needs a good diet to help them heal. Nutrition after surgery is very important for giving the body the nutrients it needs, helping tissues heal, increasing the immune system, and lowering inflammation.

A well-balanced diet full of nutrient-dense foods can help you heal faster and avoid problems as much as possible. In this in-depth guide, we'll talk about the idea of a post-surgery diet for lung surgery patients, focusing on soft, easily digestible foods for quick recovery, foods that fight inflammation and ease pain, and ways to stay hydrated that are necessary for healing after surgery.

Soft, easily digestible foods to help you get better right away:

People who have had surgery on their lungs often have trouble eating and chewing because they are sore and uncomfortable. So, adding soft, easily digestible foods to your diet is very important for quick healing. These foods are easy on the digestive system, don't take much work to eat, and give you the nutrients you need to heal. Mashed potatoes, cooked veggies, oatmeal, yogurt, scrambled eggs, smoothies, soups, and pureed fruits are all soft foods that are easy to digest. These foods have a lot of fiber, vitamins, minerals, and protein, all of which are important for keeping your health in general and helping tissues heal. Incorporating protein-rich foods like eggs, yogurt, and liquid meats can also help keep muscles strong and stop muscle loss while you're recovering.

Foods that can help reduce pain and inflammation:

Pain and inflammation are typical side effects of lung surgery that can make recovery take longer and make patients feel worse. So, eating foods that are low in inflammation can help lower pain and inflammation and speed up the healing process. Foods that are high in phytonutrients, omega-3 fatty acids, and vitamins have been shown to reduce inflammation and can help with inflammation after surgery. Some foods that can help reduce inflammation are fatty fish (like salmon and mackerel), nuts and seeds (like flaxseeds and almonds), leafy greens (like spinach and kale), berries (like blueberries and strawberries), turmeric, ginger, and green tea. These foods not only help lower inflammation, but they also give you important nutrients that help your immune system and health in general.

Ways to stay hydrated to help your body heal after surgery:

Staying hydrated is important for healing after surgery because it helps keep the body's fluid balance, supports muscle repair, and makes it easier to get rid of toxins. Dehydration can make complaints like tiredness, dizziness, and constipation worse after surgery, which slows down the healing process. So, people who have had lung surgery need to make sure they stay refreshed by drinking enough fluids throughout the day. Besides drinking water, eating foods like fruits and veggies that are high in water can also help you stay hydrated. Fruits and vegetables that keep you hydrated are watermelon, cucumber, oranges, strawberries, celery, and tomatoes. Sugary and fizzy drinks can make you dehydrated and slow down the healing process, so it's best to stay away from them. To stay properly hydrated during the recovery time after surgery, choose drinks like water, herbal teas, and electrolyte-rich drinks.

diet after surgery is very important for helping lung surgery patients heal and get better. Focusing on soft, easily digestible foods for instant recovery, adding anti-inflammatory foods to fight inflammation and ease pain, and staying properly hydrated are all things that patients can do to speed up their healing process after surgery and achieve long-term health. Talking to a registered dietitian or another health worker can also help you get personalised nutrition advice that fits your needs and makes sure your recovery goes smoothly.

CHAPTER 3
PROTEIN-RICH HEALTH RECIPES

Protein is very important for healing after surgery on the lungs. It helps damaged organs heal and grow back by giving cells, tissues, and muscles the building blocks they need. Protein is also important for building up the immune system, which is especially important during the healing process to keep you from getting sick and improve your general health. Adding protein-rich foods to your diet after surgery can help you heal faster, give you more energy, and help you get better faster.

How Protein Helps with Recovery

Nutritionally, protein is very important because it helps the body do many things, especially when it's healing. When someone has surgery on their lungs, their body needs more protein to fix damaged tissues, build muscle strength, and make their immune system work better. Protein is important for wound healing because it gives the body the amino acids it needs to make new tissue and collagen. This speed up the healing process and lowers the risk of problems like infections. Protein also helps keep lean body mass and stops muscle loss, which can happen when you can't move around for a while after surgery. By making protein-rich foods a priority in your diet after surgery, you can help your body heal better and improve your health in general.

Soups and broths that are full of protein

People who have had surgery on their lungs should eat soups and broths because they are easy to swallow and can be full of protein-rich foods. Adding lean meats like chicken, turkey, or fish to homemade soups is a great way to get a lot of high-quality protein and other important nutrients like minerals and vitamins. Soups can also get more protein by adding legumes like lentils, beans, or chickpeas.

They also add fiber, which is good for your gut system. Another healthy choice is bone broth, which is made by simmering animal bones and connective tissue. It is high in collagen and amino acids, which help fix tissues and keep joints healthy. Adding soups and broths that are high in protein to your post-surgery meal plan will give your body the nutrients it needs while also helping it heal and recover.

Smoothies and shakes with a lot of protein

Making smoothies and shakes is an easy and flexible way to get more protein while you're recovering.

By mixing Greek yogurt, protein powder, fruits, and veggies, you can make nutrient-dense drinks that are also easy to digest. This makes them perfect for people who don't want to eat much or have trouble chewing. Greek yogurt is a great way to get protein and probiotics, which are good for your gut health and immune system. Adding protein powder made from whey, soy, or pea protein can make smoothies even higher in protein without changing the way they taste or feel. Also, adding things like nut butter, chia seeds, or hemp seeds can give you good fats and extra protein to help you feel full and give you energy. Adding high-protein drinks and shakes to your daily routine can help you get enough nutrients and speed up the healing process after surgery.

Protein bowls and salads that are good for you

Protein bowls and salads are flexible and nutrient-dense options for meals after surgery. They contain protein, carbs, and healthy fats that help with recovery and general health. Protein bowls can be made with whole grains like quinoa or brown rice as the base and lean protein sources like grilled chicken, tofu, or edamame as the toppings.

The bowls should also have a range of colorful vegetables, herbs, and dressings. In the same way, making a salad with veggies, nuts, seeds, leafy greens, and a protein source like grilled salmon or hard-boiled eggs can give you the nutrients and antioxidants you need to heal and reduce inflammation. Using avocado, olive oil, or tahini-based dressings can improve the nutritional value of food while also adding flavor and healthy fats.

By eating healthy protein bowls and salads after surgery, you can give your body the nutrients it needs to heal and stay healthy in the long run.

Finally, making protein-rich foods a priority in your diet after surgery is important for helping you heal properly, regaining your strength, and improving your general health. Soups and broths that are high in protein, smoothies and shakes that are high in protein, and protein bowls and salads that are high in protein can all help your body get the nutrients it needs to heal and thrive in the long run.

Another thing that can help you customize your diet to meet your specific needs and speed up your recovery after lung surgery is talking to a doctor or trained dietitian.

CHAPTER 4

POWERHOUSES FOR VITAMINS AND MINERALS

How Vitamins and Minerals Help the Body Heal:

You can't say enough good things about vitamins and minerals when it comes to healing after surgery. These important nutrients are very important for the body's healing processes because they help repair tissues, keep the immune system healthy, and keep the body healthy generally. Vitamins like C, A, and E are known to be antioxidants. Antioxidants help lower inflammation and oxidative stress, which speeds up the mending process. Minerals like magnesium, calcium, and zinc are also important for keeping bones healthy and muscles working well, which are both important for healing. Vitamins B complex, which includes B6 and B12, are also important for making energy and keeping nerves working properly, which boosts general health during the healing process.

Smoothies and juices full of vitamins:

Smoothies and drinks that are high in vitamins are one of the easiest and most effective ways to add vitamins to your diet after surgery. Not only are these drinks cool, but they are also full of healthy nutrients that help the body heal. Oranges, lemons, berries (blueberries, strawberries), tropical fruits (pineapples, mangoes), and leafy greens (spinach, kale) are all great foods that are high in antioxidants and vitamins C and A. Putting in things like yogurt or nut milk gives these drinks more calcium and protein, making them even healthier. Adding flaxseeds or chia seeds also increases the amount of omega-3 fatty acids, which help reduce inflammation. Drinking these vitamin-rich drinks every day can help the body heal faster and stay healthy generally.

Vegetable and grain bowls that are high in nutrients:

Having nutrient-dense veggie and grain bowls after surgery is another great way to make sure you get enough vitamins and minerals. Not only do these meals make you feel full, but they also give you a lot of nutrients that your body needs to heal.

To begin, use whole grains like quinoa, brown rice, or barley as your base. These foods are full of fiber, vitamins, and minerals. Then, add a variety of colorful veggies, like broccoli, carrots, bell peppers, and leafy greens. These vegetables are good for you because they contain antioxidants, phytonutrients, and vitamins A, C, and K. Adding lean protein sources like grilled chicken, tofu, or beans to your diet gives your body the amino acids it needs to repair tissues and keep muscles in good shape.

Add healthy herbs and spices to the bowl, like turmeric, ginger, garlic, and parsley, to make it taste better and give it more nutrients. These herbs and spices are known to reduce inflammation and boost the immune system. Trying out different combinations of ingredients is the best way to make sure you have a varied, nutrient-rich diet that helps you heal and stay healthy in the long run.

Herbs and spices that are good for you can be used in tasty ways:

Herbs and spices not only make food taste better, but they are also good for you in many ways, so they should be an important part of your diet after surgery. Adding healing spices and plants to food not only makes it taste better but also gives you extra nutrients and medical benefits that help you get better. For example, curcumin, which is found in turmeric, is a strong anti-inflammatory and antioxidant that can help lessen pain and swelling after surgery. Ginger is another vegetable that is known to help with nausea and reduce inflammation, which makes it especially helpful for people who have recently had surgery. Onions and garlic have a lot of sulfur compounds that help the immune system work and clean out the body, which speeds up the mending process. Some other helpful herbs and spices are celery, which is high in vitamins C and K, which are needed for bone health and wound healing, and cinnamon, which helps keep blood sugar levels steady. Adding these healing herbs and spices to stews, soups, stir-fries, and marinades not only makes the food taste better but also gives you extra nutrients to help you recover from surgery and stay healthy in the long run.

CHAPTER 5

MEALS HIGH IN ANTIOXIDANTS FOR GOOD RESPIRATORY HEALTH

Before getting into specific recipes and meal plans designed to help lung surgery patients recover as quickly as possible, it's important to understand how vitamins help keep the lungs healthy. Antioxidants are chemicals that can be found in many foods. They help get rid of free radicals, which are dangerous molecules that can damage cells, including those in the respiratory system. Making sure that people who have recently had surgery on their lungs eat a lot of antioxidant-rich foods can help reduce inflammation, boost their immune systems, and speed up their general healing.

How to Understand How Important Antioxidants Are

Antioxidants are very important for lung health because they keep lung cells from getting hurt by inflammation and oxidative stress. The lungs are especially sensitive to oxidative damage because they are constantly exposed to irritants, allergens, and pollutants in the environment.

These outside factors can cause free radicals, which can cause inflammation and tissue damage.

This can make breathing problems worse and slow down the healing process after surgery. By getting rid of free radicals and lowering reactive stress, antioxidants help reduce inflammation, boost the immune system, and help lung tissue heal.

Bright salads that are full of antioxidant-rich goodness

Including colorful veggies in your meal plans after surgery can be a great way to get more antioxidants and nutrients that your body needs to heal. Flavonoids, vitamin C, vitamin E, and beta-carotene are found in large amounts in leafy greens like spinach, kale, and rocket.

Adding colorful veggies to salads, like broccoli, bell pepper, tomatoes, and carrots, makes them even higher in antioxidants. Adding nuts, seeds, and avocado to salads not only changes the taste and texture but also adds healthy fats and more vitamins. Adding dressings made from olive oil, lemon juice, and plants that are high in antioxidants can make salads even healthier.

This makes them a great choice for supporting lung health while you recover.

Skillets and stir-fries that boost the immune system

Stir-fries and pan meals are easy and tasty ways to add antioxidant-rich foods to your diet after surgery to help your immune system work better. Bell pepper, broccoli, carrots, and snap peas are some of the colorful veggies that go well in stir-fry. They are full of antioxidants, vitamins, and minerals that your body needs to heal.

Adding lean proteins like fish, chicken, tofu, or eggs not only gives you important nutrients but also helps your body heal and fix itself. Adding immune-boosting herbs and spices like oregano, ginger, turmeric, and garlic to stir-fries not only makes them taste better but also helps fight inflammation and free radicals. Whole grains, like brown rice or quinoa, added to stir-fries give you more fiber and complex carbs, which help your energy and general health while you're healing.

Snacks and sides that are full of flavor and antioxidants

Along with main meals, eating tasty snacks and sides that are high in vitamins can help your lungs stay healthy and speed up the healing process after surgery. Berries, citrus fruits, and kiwis are great snacks for people who have had lung surgery because they are high in vitamin C and other antioxidants. Fruits and nuts or yogurt together make a balanced and enjoyable snack because the nuts or yogurt add protein and healthy fats. Herbs and spices added to roasted veggies make them taste great and fill you up. They are also full of antioxidants and nutrients that your body needs to heal. Adding antioxidant-rich dips and spreads like guacamole, olive tapenade, or hummus to snacks and sides can make them even healthier while also making the diet more interesting and varied after surgery.

Finally, eating foods that are high in antioxidants is very important for people who have recently had surgery to help their bodies heal properly and keep their lungs healthy. Lung surgery patients can give their bodies the nutrients they need for recovery and long-term health by learning about the value of antioxidants and eating colourful salads, immune-boosting stir-fries, and tasty snacks and sides. People can start improving their respiratory health and general well-being by focusing on whole, nutrient-dense foods and tasty recipes that are designed to help the body heal.

CHAPTER 6

SOUPS THAT WILL COMFORT AND HEAL YOU

People have long said that soups are comfort foods because they keep you warm and feed your soul. This is especially true for people who have recently had surgery and are still recovering. Soups are soothing, they can help your body digest food, they contain important nutrients, and they are a gentle way to recover after surgery. The next part talks about how soups can help you heal. It includes both traditional soup recipes and new ones that are perfect for a post-surgery diet.

How Soups Can Help You Feel Better During Recovery

Having surgery, no matter what kind, can be hard on the body. During the healing process, it is very important to eat foods that help the body heal and are good for general health. Thus, soups become a particularly good choice because they are easy to digest and gently give important nutrients.

Soup can also help people who are in pain or discomfort after surgery because it is warm. Soups are also flexible enough to fit specific dietary needs or tastes, which makes them a good choice for people who are still recovering. Soups come in many forms, from clear broths to hearty stews, and can be used in many ways to heal and feed.

Classic and unique soup recipes

When it comes to nutrition after surgery, basic soup recipes stand out because they are easy to make and work well. For example, chicken noodle soup is famous for making people feel better and possibly even helping their defense systems. This classic food is full of protein, vitamins, and minerals that can help your body repair itself and give you more energy. In the same way, vegetable soup is full of healthy nutrients like fiber, vitamins, and phytonutrients that help the body heal and stay healthy.

In addition to these classic choices, creative soup recipes let you try new tastes and ingredients while still following the rules of healthy eating after surgery. For example, ginger and turmeric added to creamy butternut squash soup can help reduce inflammation and make the taste more interesting. Adding fragrant spices like cumin and coriander to lentil soup makes it taste great.

 It also has a lot of plant-based protein and fiber, which helps your stomach and makes you feel full. Both basic and creative soup recipes can help you eat well after surgery by using a variety of ingredients that are good for you and help you heal.

Broths and stews that are good for your body and soul

Broths and stews are not only tasty, but they are also very good for you when you are recovering from surgery.

It is thought that clear broths, like bone broth or veggie broth, are very healthy and easy for the body to absorb. Being full of minerals, amino acids, and collagen, bone broth is a highly sought-after healing potion that helps the gut stay healthy, joints work well, and the immune system stays strong.

In the same way, veggie broths are full of vitamins, minerals, and antioxidants that help the body's defenses and heal damaged tissues. Stews have a hearty texture and a strong flavor. They also contain a lot of protein and other important nutrients that help repair muscles and speed up healing in general. Stews are a comforting and healthy food choice for people who have recently had surgery. They can be made with tender cuts of meat or a variety of seasonal veggies. By including broths and stews in their diet after surgery, people can use the healing properties of these common foods to help them recover quickly and stay healthy in the long run.

CHAPTER 7

GRAINS AND CARBOHYDRATES THAT ARE EASY TO DIGEST

It's impossible to say enough about how important easy-to-digest grains and carbs are for healing after surgery. When someone has surgery on their lungs, their body goes through a lot of stress and needs a lot of nutrients to help them heal.

Of these necessary nutrients, carbohydrates are very important because they give the body energy and help repair damaged tissues. But not all starches are the same, especially when it comes to recovering from surgery.

Here, we talk about how important it is to choose the right carbohydrates, look at some easy and filling rice and grain meals, and talk about how soft and comforting bread and pasta are as important parts of a complete diet after surgery.

How to Choose the Best Carbs for Recovery

People who are healing from lung surgery need to make sure they eat the right carbohydrates. Choosing types that are easy to digest can help keep stomach pain to a minimum and improve nutrient absorption.

Whole grains like oats, brown rice, and quinoa are great options because they have a lot of fiber, which helps your body digest food and gives you energy that lasts.

Furthermore, refined carbs such as white rice and pasta may be easier on the digestive system at first, especially right after surgery when digestion may be weak.

Whole grains, on the other hand, should always be chosen over refined carbs because they have better nutrition. Including a range of food sources also makes sure you get a wide range of important nutrients, which is good for your health and well-being while you're recovering.

Simple and tasty grain and rice dishes

Rice and grain foods can be used in many ways to make healthy meals that are good for recovering from surgery. Simple dishes like steamed rice or quinoa are great for people with sensitive digestive systems because they have a neutral base that goes well with many types of proteins and veggies. Adding herbs and spices not only makes food taste better, but they may also help with digestion and reduce inflammation.

For instance, ginger and turmeric are naturally anti-inflammatory, which can help reduce pain and swelling after surgery. Adding cooked veggies like bell peppers, carrots, and spinach to these dishes boosts their nutritional value by adding fiber, vitamins, and minerals that help the body heal.

Adding protein sources like tofu, chicken, or fish to your diet also makes sure you get enough of the important amino acids your body needs to repair tissues and keep your immune system healthy.

Bread and pasta that are soft and comforting

Because they are soft and comforting, bread and pasta are an easy way to get more carbs while also feeling good during the recovery time. Instead of white bread and pasta, choose whole-grain versions whenever you can. They have more fiber, vitamins, and minerals.

But people whose digestion isn't working well may find refined types easier to handle at first. Toasted whole grain bread spread with avocado or nut butter is a healthy snack that is high in nutrients and healthy fats, which are needed to fix cells and control inflammation.

In the same way, adding whole-grain pasta to soups or casseroles gives meals more texture and depth while giving you a healthy dose of carbs. Trying gluten-free options like brown rice pasta or chickpea flour bread can work around dietary rules while still giving you the nutrients you need for a quick recovery.

adding easy-to-digest carbs and grains to your diet after surgery is very important for speeding up recovery and maintaining long-term health. People can support their recovery while having tasty and healthy meals by choosing the right carbohydrates, like whole grains, and adding them to simple, filling dishes. Bread and pasta that are soft and cozy are other ways to get more carbs while also feeling better and giving you more options while you heal. In the end, eating nutrient-dense foods first and sticking to a healthy diet that is tailored to your needs are two of the most important things you can do to improve your health after surgery and keep it up.

CHAPTER 8

BEVERAGES THAT HEALTH AND HYDRATE

Getting enough water is very important for getting better after lung surgery. The body needs a lot of fluids to keep itself healthy, help cells work, and speed up the repair process. In this part, we'll talk about how important it is to stay hydrated during recovery, look at the health benefits of herbal teas and infusions, and stress how important it is to eat smoothies and juices after surgery.

How important it is to stay hydrated during recovery

People who are having lung treatment need to make sure they stay hydrated because it helps the body's natural healing processes and prevents problems. Surgery and anesthesia can make you dehydrated, which can make complaints like fatigue, dizziness, and constipation worse after surgery.

Staying hydrated helps the blood flow, which brings oxygen and nutrients to cells and makes them easier to heal and grow back. Also, staying hydrated helps thin the mucus that forms in the lungs, which makes it easier to clear out and lowers the risk of respiratory problems like asthma.

To help their healing and get the best results, patients should try to drink a lot of fluids, such as water, herbal teas, and other hydrating drinks.

Herbal teas and infusions that are good for you

Adding herbal teas and refreshing liquids to your diet after surgery can help you stay hydrated and heal at the same time. Herbal teas, like peppermint, chamomile, and ginger, are full of anti-inflammatory and antioxidant chemicals that can help ease pain after surgery and speed up the healing process. Chamomile tea in particular is known for its ability to calm people down. It can help people relax and sleep, which are both very important for healing. Anti-nausea features in ginger tea make it helpful for people who are feeling sick after surgery and throwing up.

Having digestive problems and bloating after surgery is normal. Peppermint tea can help ease these symptoms. Herbal infusions, such as lemon and honey water, also help you stay hydrated while boosting your immune system and supporting your general health. Adding these soothing drinks to your diet after surgery can help you stay hydrated and heal from the inside out.

Smoothies and juices that hydrate

Fruit and vegetable shakes and juices are easy and tasty ways to drink more water and give your body the nutrients it needs. Smoothies made with fresh fruits, veggies, and coconut water are a great way to stay hydrated. They are also a great source of vitamins, minerals, and antioxidants that help the body heal and fight off illness.

Adding leafy veggies like spinach and kale to smoothies can make them more nutritious and help the body heal itself. Adding protein-rich foods like Greek yogurt or plant-based protein powder can help your muscles recover and wounds heal faster. In the same way, freshly squeezed juices made from different fruits and veggies can be a concentrated source of nutrients and water.

The anti-inflammatory and detoxifying qualities of carrot, beetroot, and celery juice make them especially helpful for helping the body heal and reducing inflammation after surgery. Adding smoothies and juices that are high in water to your diet after surgery can help replace lost electrolytes, keep you hydrated, and improve your general health while you heal.

staying properly hydrated is very important for speedy healing after lung surgery. Adding herbal teas, smoothies, juices, and other refreshing drinks to your diet after surgery can help you heal and stay healthy in the long run.

Plus, they contain therapeutic compounds that can help your body heal. Individuals can speed up their recovery and have better results after lung surgery by prioritizing staying hydrated and adding these healing drinks to their diet.

CHAPTER 9

SNACKS AND TREATS TO KEEP YOU HEALTHY AND HAPPY

As someone recovers from lung surgery, eating a healthy diet is very important to help them get better. Improving your nutrition is very important for speeding up the healing process because it gives your body the nutrients it needs for tissue repair, immune system function, and general health.

A post-surgery diet should mostly consist of meals, but adding snacks and treats can not only help you stay healthy, but they can also bring you joy and comfort while you're healing.

Ideas for healthy snacks that will keep you going:

When it comes to eating after surgery, choosing healthy snacks is important to keep your energy up and help your body heal.

As much as possible, these snacks should be full of healthy fats, vitamins, minerals, protein, and other nutrients that are important for the body's healing. By eating a range of nutrient-dense foods, patients can make sure they get all the nutrients they need, which helps them get back to their best health after surgery. Fresh fruits like oranges, berries, and apples are good healthy snacks for people who have recently had surgery on their lungs because they are full of vitamins, enzymes, and fiber, which help the immune system and digestion.

Adding nuts and seeds, like pumpkin seeds, walnuts, and almonds, can also give you protein, healthy fats, and micronutrients that your body needs to mend and maintain tissues.

Greek yogurt with honey and granola is a healthy and filling snack that provides probiotics for gut health, protein for muscle repair, and carbs for long-lasting energy. Having hummus with whole grain crackers or vegetable sticks gives you a healthy mix of protein, fiber, and healthy fats, which helps you feel full and keeps your digestive system healthy. Also, avocado toast on whole-grain bread is a healthy food full of heart-healthy fats, fiber, and vitamins that help reduce inflammation and speed up the healing of tissues. Adding these healthy snacks to your diet after surgery will not only help your body heal, but it will also improve your general health and vitality.

Indulgent treats to make you feel better:

Prioritizing nutrient-dense snacks is important for a speedy recovery, but sweet treats can also help lift your mood and make the whole experience better after surgery.

It is important to find a balance between treats and nutrients by making sure that treats are eaten in moderation and that a mostly healthy diet is also followed.

 Indulgent treats can bring you joy and comfort while you're healing, which is good for your mental health and emotional strength.

With its strong flavor and antioxidants, dark chocolate can be enjoyed in moderation as a sweet treat that might also be good for your heart and make you feel better. Also, fresh baked goods like oatmeal cookies or banana bread made with healthy ingredients like nuts, bananas, and oats can be a comforting treat while still giving you the fiber and nutrients you need.

Frozen yogurt or sorbet made with natural sweeteners and fresh fruits is a tasty treat that you can enjoy without feeling guilty. It's great for filling your sweet tooth and staying hydrated while also providing nutrients. It's important to enjoy treats in balance and with awareness, savoring each bite and watching how much you eat to avoid eating too many unhealthy fats and refined sugars.

As long as people include things that aren't healthy in moderation in their diet after surgery, they can feel good about themselves and enjoy life without hurting their health or well-being.

Energy bars and bites made at home:

People who have recently had surgery on their lungs can make their energy bars and bites as easy and healthy snacks to help their bodies heal. Commercially made energy bars may have added sugars, preservatives, and artificial ingredients.

Homemade versions, on the other hand, can be made to fit each person's tastes and nutritional needs by using only natural, healthy ingredients. People can make sure that the quality and amount of ingredients in their energy bars and bites are in line with their health goals and personal tastes by making them at home.

Oats, nuts, seeds, and dried fruits are all great base ingredients for making your energy bars. They are full of complex carbs, protein, healthy fats, and micronutrients that your body needs for long-lasting energy and muscle repair. Using natural sweeteners like honey or maple syrup makes the food taste better and helps the body get carbs and energy back.

Making homemade energy bars taste better and healthier by adding things like nut butter, coconut oil, and cocoa powder gives them more depth and flavor.

 People can make homemade energy bars that fit their taste preferences and dietary needs by trying out different flavor combinations and textures.

This makes them a tasty and satisfying snack choice for recovering from surgery.

Also, dividing energy bars into single pieces and keeping them in an airtight container makes it easy to get healthy snacks throughout the day, which can help control your energy and hunger. Homemade energy bars and bites are a handy and healthy way for people who want to improve their recovery from lung surgery while still satisfying their cravings for healthy and tasty snacks. They can be eaten as a pre-workout boost, a midday pick-me-up, or a treat after dinner.

CHAPTER 10
TALKS ABOUT LONG-TERM RECOVERY AND MAINTENANCE.

After having surgery on the lungs, one of the most important parts of the healing process is long-term care and recovery. This phase is about switching to normal eating habits, making sure those habits will last for a long time, and continuing to support lung health through nutrition. Each part is very important for a faster recovery after surgery, better health in general, and a lower chance of complications.

Getting used to regular eating habits

Getting back to normal eating habits after lung surgery is a slow process that needs careful planning of food choices and times. At first, people may have changes in their hunger, stomach pain, and limitations on certain foods.

As the healing process goes on, though, it's important to start eating a varied diet full of nutrient-rich foods again to help the body heal and stay healthy.

One part of getting back to regular eating is slowly adding solid foods again while keeping an eye on tolerance levels. Start with foods that are easy to digest, like soups, broths, and soft fruits.

Then add in more complicated foods, like vegetables, lean proteins, and whole grains, over time. To avoid pain or problems, it is important to pay attention to your body's signals and make changes to your food as needed.

Hydration is another important thing to think about during this time. Getting enough fluids is important for keeping your health in general, helping you heal, and keeping you from becoming dehydrated. Aim to drink a lot of water throughout the day, and think about eating foods that are high in water, like fruits, veggies, and herbal teas.

Long-Term Healthy Eating Habits That You Can Keep Up

Setting up healthy eating habits that last is important for long-term health and happiness after lung surgery. Eating a balanced, varied diet with lots of different nutrients can help your body heal, improve your immune system, and lower your risk of complications. Whole, nutrient-dense foods like fruits, veggies, lean proteins, whole grains, and healthy fats should be a big part of your meals.

Eating a range of fruits and veggies gives you important vitamins, minerals, and antioxidants that are good for your lungs and your overall health. Aim to eat a wide range of colorful fruits and veggies to get the most nutrients and help your body heal. Also, to help your muscles heal and fix, choose lean protein sources like chicken, fish, beans, and tofu.

Whole grains, like brown rice, quinoa, oats, and whole wheat, are full of fiber, vitamins, and minerals that are good for your digestive system and give you the energy that lasts.

Adding these foods to your diet can help keep your blood sugar levels in check, help you control your weight, and lower your risk of getting chronic diseases.

Keeping up good nutrition for lung health

For long-term health and a lower chance of respiratory problems, it's important to eat well and keep your lungs healthy. Vitamin C, vitamin E, beta-carotene, and omega-3 fatty acids are some of the nutrients that have been shown to help the lungs work better, lower inflammation, and boost the immune system.

Citrus fruits, strawberries, kiwis, and bell peppers are all high in vitamin C, which can help protect against respiratory infections and help your body make collagen, which helps fix tissues. Vitamin E can be found in nuts, seeds, and veggie oils.

It is an antioxidant that keeps lung cells from getting damaged by free radicals.

Beta-carotene is found in orange and yellow fruits and veggies like squash, carrots, and sweet potatoes. It is turned into vitamin A in the body and helps keep the lungs healthy and the immune system working well. Adding these foods to your diet can help keep your lungs healthy and lower your risk of getting lung-related problems.

Omega-3 fatty acids can be found in flaxseeds, chia seeds, walnuts, and fatty fish. They can help reduce inflammation in the lungs and improve respiratory health generally. Lung diseases like asthma, chronic obstructive pulmonary disease (COPD), and bronchitis are less likely to happen if you eat these things.

Along with certain nutrients, lung health needs to stay at a healthy weight by eating well and exercising regularly. Being overweight can put stress on the lungs and make breathing problems worse, so keeping a healthy weight can help your lungs work better and your general health.

Following a nutrient-dense diet with a range of fruits, veggies, lean proteins, whole grains, and healthy fats can help with long-term recovery and maintenance after lung surgery. You can improve your lung health, lower your chance of complications, and support your overall health for years to come by eating these foods and making them a regular part of your diet.

CONCLUSION

For those who are starting on this road, this complete guide has lit the way to the best post-surgery diet, giving them hope and healing.

From pre-surgery preparation, which includes eating right and eating foods that boost your immune system, to post-surgery essentials, which include eating foods that are easy for your body to digest and staying hydrated to speed up the healing process, each chapter has been carefully written to help you through every step of your recovery.

The focus on protein-rich foods, meals high in vitamins and minerals, and meals high in antioxidants shows how important nutrients are for healing and improving lung health. Soups that make you feel better, grains that are easy to handle, and drinks that keep you hydrated are all good for you while you're healing.

As we talk about long-term recovery and upkeep, this guide goes beyond just healing you right now. It gives you advice on how to keep your health and support for lung wellness going for a long time.

In the end, this guide isn't just a collection of recipes; it's also a demonstration of how nutrition can help build resilience, energy, and long-term health. May it be a reliable guide on your way to recovery and success after surgery, leading you to a future full of health, vigor, and happiness.

www.ingramcontent.com/pod-product-compliance
Lightning Source LLC
Chambersburg PA
CBHW070319290526
45791CB00003B/1172